Quick and Easy Dash Diet

A collection of Delicacies to stay Healthy and Fit perfect for busy People

Natalie Puckett

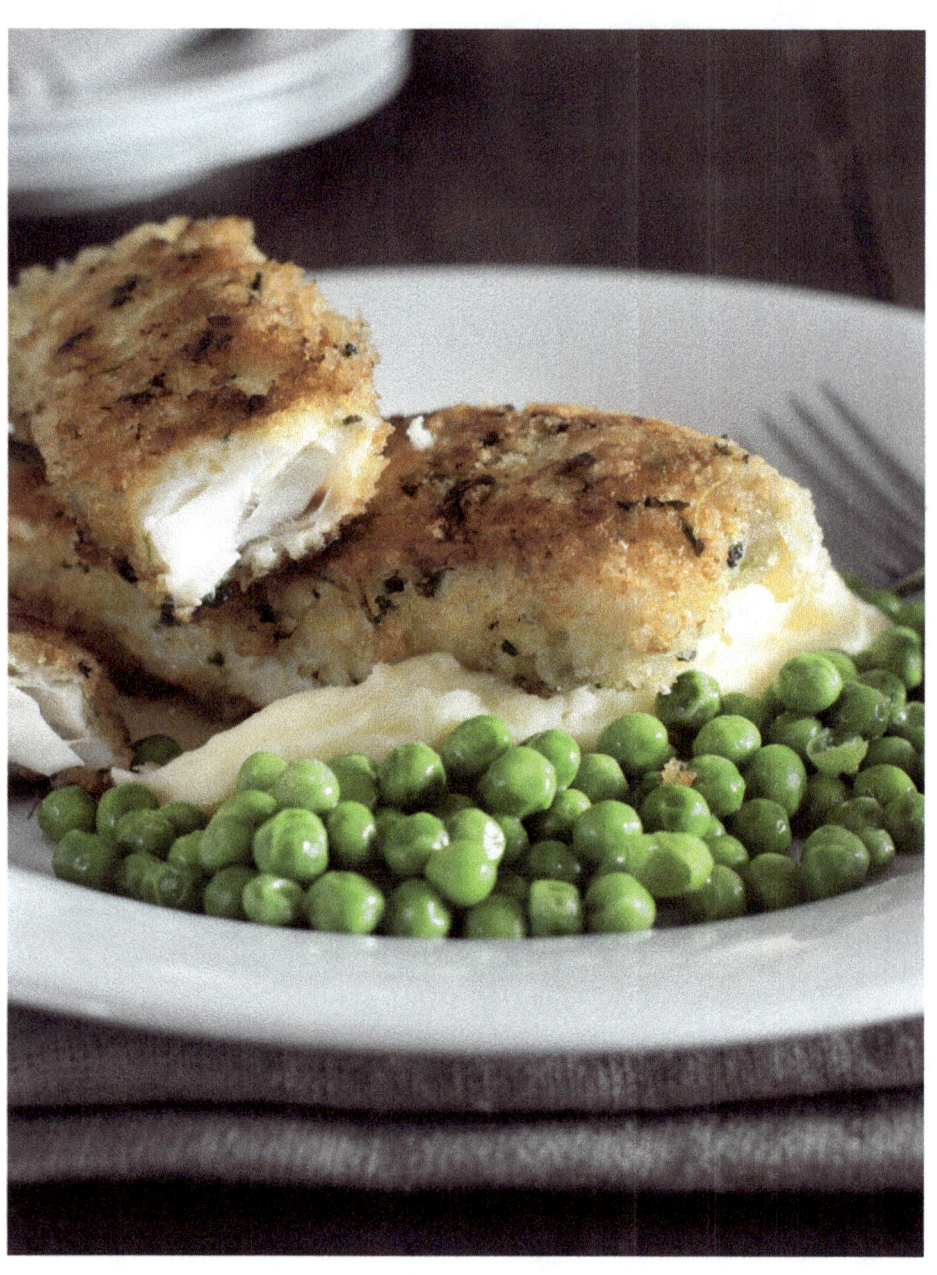

© copyright 2021 – all rights reserved.

the content contained within this book may not be reproduced, duplicated or transmitted without direct written permission from the author or the publisher.

under no circumstances will any blame or legal responsibility be held against the publisher, or author, for any damages, reparation, or monetary loss due to the information contained within this book. either directly or indirectly.

legal notice:

this book is copyright protected. this book is only for personal use. you cannot amend, distribute, sell, use, quote or paraphrase any part, or the content within this book, without the consent of the author or publisher.

disclaimer notice:

please note the information contained within this document is for educational and entertainment purposes only. all effort has been executed to present accurate, up to date, and reliable, complete information. no warranties of any kind are declared or implied. readers acknowledge that the author is not engaging in the rendering of legal, financial, medical or professional advice. the content within this book has been derived from various sources. please consult a licensed professional before attempting any techniques outlined in this book.

by reading this document, the reader agrees that under no circumstances is the author responsible for any losses, direct or indirect, which are incurred as a result of the use of information contained within this document, including, but not limited to, ― errors, omissions, or inaccuracies.

Table of Contents

HERB-CRUSTED BAKED COD 5
SHRIMP KEBABS 7
ROASTED SALMON 9
SHRIMP WITH CORN HASH 11
SHRIMP CEVICHE 14
REFRESHING WATERMELON SORBET 16
LOVELY FAUX MAC AND CHEESE 18
BEAUTIFUL BANANA CUSTARD 20
HEALTHY TAHINI BUNS 23
SPICY PECAN BOWL 25
GENTLE SWEET POTATO TEMPURA 27
JAPANESE CUCUMBER SUNOMONO 30
RADISH AND HASH BROWN DISH 32
KID FRIENDLY POPSICLES 34
THE PEAR AND CHOCOLATE CATASTROPHE 36
THE AVOCADO PARADISE 38
THE AUTHENTIC VEGETABLE MEDLEY 40
THE ORIGINAL POWER PRODUCER 42
THE DREAMY CHERRY MIX 44
LEMON SMOOTHIE 46
ONE THE WATERMELON 49
STRAWBERRY AND RHUBARB SMOOTHIE 51
DECISIVE CAULIFLOWER AND MUSHROOM RISOTTO 53
AUTHENTIC ZUCCHINI BOATS 55
ROASTED ONIONS AND GREEN BEANS 57
SUGAR BREAK APPLE AND PEANUT BUTTER OATMEAL 60
SWEET POTATO TOAST 62
GRANELLI 63
TOFU TURMERIC SCRAMBLE 65

- Whole Grain Cheese Pancakes 67
- Red Pepper, Kale, and Cheddar Frittata 70
- Scrambled Eggs with Bell Pepper and Feta 72
- Devilled Egg Toast 73
- Basic Scrambled Eggs 74
- Baked Butternut-Squash Rigatoni 77
- Simple Caprese Sandwich 79
- Cottage Cheese Honey Toast 80
- Pimento Cheese Sandwich 81
- Tomato Salad 82
- Tomato and Cheese Wrap 84
- Peanut Butter Yogurt 86
- Peanut Butter & Carrots 88
- Cucumber Tomato Salad with Tuna 89
- Peanut butter and Jelly 90
- Chicken Scampi Pasta 92
- Apple-Cherry Pork Medallions 94
- Butternut Turkey Soup 96
- Black Bean & Sweet Potato Rice Bowls 98
- Pepper Ricotta Primavera 101
- Bow Ties with Sausage & Asparagus 103

Herb-Crusted Baked Cod

Prep time: 10 minutes

Cook time: 10 minutes

Servings: 4

Ingredients

Herb-flavored stuffing – ¾ cup, crushed until crumbed

Cod fillets – 4 (4 ounces each)

Honey - ¼ cup

Method

1. Preheat the oven to 375F. Coat a baking pan with cooking spray.

2. Brush the fillets with honey. Discard the rest of the honey.

3. Place the stuffing in a bag and place a fillet in the bag.

4. Shake the bag to coat the cod well.

5. Remove the fillet and repeat with the remaining fillets.

Bake the fillets for 10 minutes or until opaque throughout.

Nutritional Facts Per Serving

Calories: 185

Fat: 1g

Carb: 23g

Protein: 21g

Sodium 163mg

Shrimp Kebabs

Prep time: 10 minutes

Cook time: 5 minutes

Servings: 2

Ingredients

Lemon – 1, juiced

Olive oil – 1 Tbsp.

Finely minced garlic – 2 tsp.

Finely chopped fresh tarragon – 1 tsp.

Finely chopped fresh rosemary – 1 tsp.

Kosher salt - ½ tsp.

Ground black pepper – ¼ tsp.

Shrimp – 12 pieces, peeled and deveined

Method

Soak 2 wooden skewers for 10 minutes.

1. Preheat grill on high.

2. In a bowl, combine seasonings, herbs, garlic, olive oil, and lemon juice.

3. Marinade the shrimp into the lemon marinade for 5 minutes.

4. Skewer the shrimp.

5. Then place on the grill. Cook until shrimp is thoroughly cooked, about 2 minutes per side.

6. Serve.

Nutritional Facts Per Serving

Calories: 105

Fat: 1g

Carb: 0g

Protein: 24g

Sodium 185mg

Roasted Salmon

Prep time: 5 minutes

Cook time: 12 minutes

Servings: 2

Ingredients

Salmon with skin – 2 (5-ounce) pieces

Extra-virgin olive oil – 2 tsp.

Chopped chives – 1 Tbsp.

Fresh tarragon leaves – 1 Tbsp.

Method

1. Preheat the oven to 425F. Line a baking sheet with foil.

2. Rub salmon with oil.

3. Line a baking sheet with foil.

4.   Place salmon (skin side down).

5.   Cook for 12 minutes or until fish is cooked through. Check after 10 minutes.

6.   Serve the salmon with herbs.

Nutritional Facts Per Serving

Calories: 244

Fat: 14g

Carb: 0g

Protein: 28g

Sodium 62mg

Shrimp with Corn Hash

Prep time: 5 minutes

Cook time: 10 minutes

Servings: 4

Ingredients

Olive oil – 4 tsp.

Large shrimp - 1 pound, peeled and deveined

Chopped red onion – ½ cup

Red bell pepper – ½, chopped

Fresh corn kernels – 1 ½ cup

Halved cherry – 1 cup

Crushed hot red pepper – ¼ tsp.

Water – ¼ cup Fresh lemon juice – 1 Tbsp.

Chopped fresh basil – 2 Tbsp.

Method

1. Heat 2 tsp. oil in a skillet.
2. Add the shrimp
3. Cook for 3 to 5 minutes. Transfer to a plate.
4. Heat remaining 2 tsp. oil in the skillet. Add bell pepper.
5. Then onion and stir-fry for 1 minute, or until softened.
6. Add tomatoes, corn, and hot pepper and cover.
7. Cook for 3 minutes.
8. Add the shrimp and reheat, stirring often, about 1 minute.
9. Stir in lemon juice and water and cook.
10. Sprinkle with basil and serve.

Nutritional Facts Per Serving

Calories: 195

Fat: 6g

Carb: 18g

Protein: 18g

Sodium 647mg

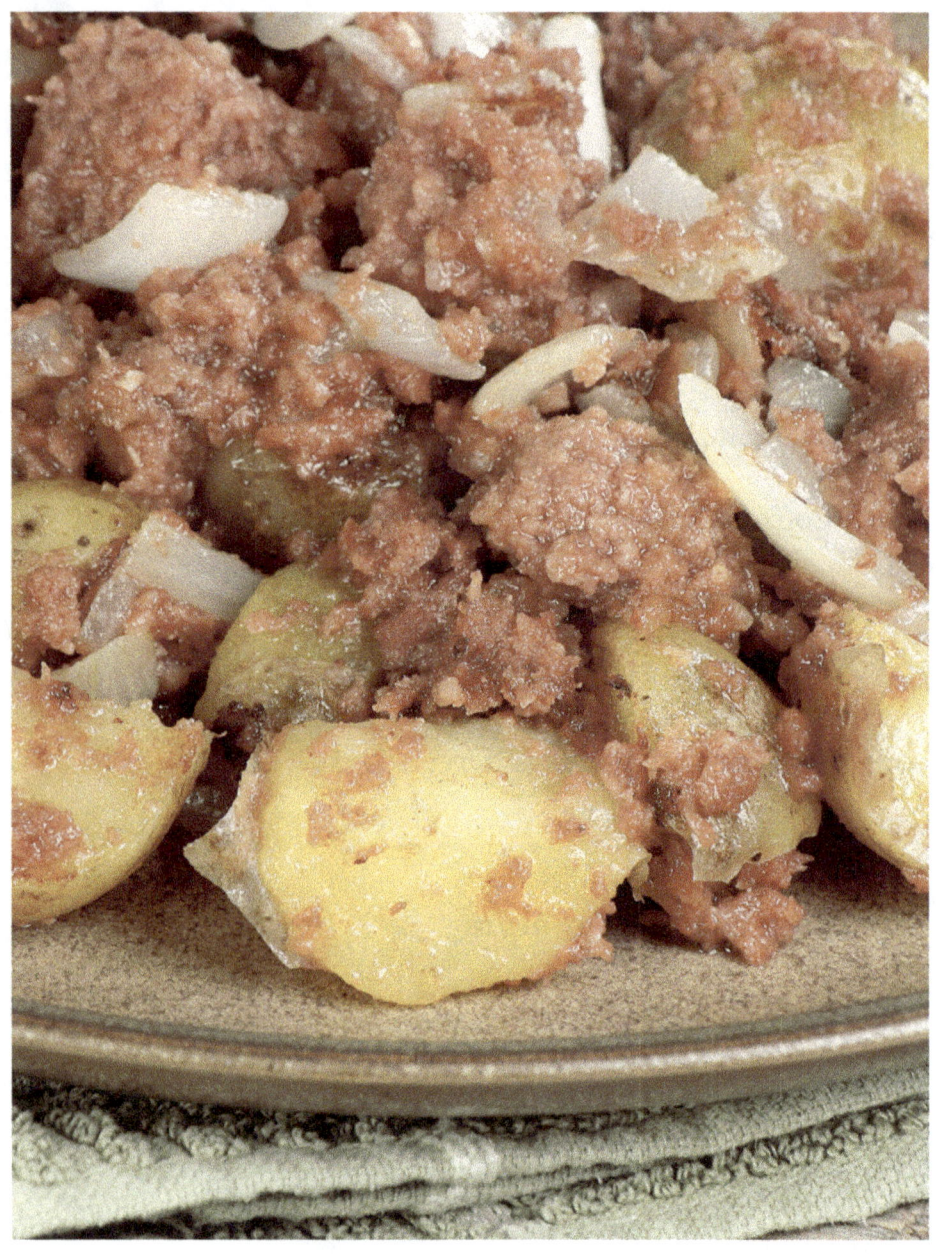

Shrimp Ceviche

Prep time: 10 minutes

Cook time: 0 minutes

Servings: 8

Ingredients

Raw shrimp – ½ pound, cut into ¼ inch pieces

Lemons – 2, zest and juice

Limes -2, zest and juice

Olive oil - 2 Tbsp.

Cumin – 2 tsp.

Diced red onion – ½ cup

Diced tomato – 1 cup

Minced garlic – 2 Tbsp.

Black beans - 1 cup, cooked

Diced serrano chili pepper – ¼ cup, seeds removed

Diced cucumber – 1 cup, peeled and seeded

Chopped cilantro – ¼ cup

Method

1. In a bowl, place the shrimp and cover with the lemon and lime juice. Marinate for at least 3 hours.

2. In another bowl, mix the remaining ingredients and set aside.

3. Before serving, mix shrimp and the juice with remaining ingredients.

4. Serve.

Nutritional Facts Per Serving

Calories: 98

Fat: 4g

Carb: 10g

Protein: 7g

Sodium 167mg

Refreshing Watermelon Sorbet

Serving: 4

Prep Time: 20 minutes + 20 hours chill time

Cook Time: Nil

Ingredients:

4 cups watermelon, seedless and chunked ¼ cup coconut sugar

2 tablespoons lime juice

How To:

1. Add the listed ingredients to a blender and puree.

2. Transfer to a freezer container with a tight-fitting lid.

3. Freeze the mix for about 4-6 hours until you have gelatin-like consistency.

4. Puree the mix once again in batches and return to the container.

5. Chill overnight.

6.   Allow the sorbet to stand for 5 minutes before serving and enjoy!

Nutrition (Per Serving)

Calories: 91

Fat: 0g

Carbohydrates: 25g

Protein: 1g

Lovely Faux Mac and Cheese

Serving: 4

Prep Time: 15 minutes

Cook Time: 45 minutes

Ingredients:

5 cups cauliflower florets

Salt and pepper to taste

1 cup coconut milk

½ cup vegetable broth

2 tablespoons coconut flour, sifted

1 organic egg, beaten

2 cups cheddar cheese

How To:

1. Pre-heat your oven to 350 degrees F.

2. Season florets with salt and steam until firm.

3. Place florets in greased ovenproof dish.

4. Heat coconut milk over medium heat in a skillet, make sure to season the oil with salt and pepper.

5. Stir in broth and add coconut flour to the mix, stir.

6. Cook until the sauce begins to bubble.

7. Remove heat and add beaten egg.

8. Pour the thick sauce over cauliflower and mix in cheese.

9. Bake for 30-45 minutes.

10. Serve and enjoy!

Nutrition (Per Serving)

Calories: 229

Fat: 14g

Carbohydrates: 9g

Protein: 15g

Beautiful Banana Custard

Serving: 3

Prep Time: 10 minutes

Cook Time: 25 minutes

Ingredients:

2 ripe bananas, peeled and mashed finely ½ teaspoon of vanilla extract

14-ounce unsweetened almond milk

3 eggs

How To:

1. Pre-heat your oven to 350 degrees F.

2. Grease 8 custard glasses lightly.

3. Arrange the glasses in a large baking dish.

4. Take a large bowl and mix all of the ingredients and mix

them well until combined nicely.

5. Divide the mixture evenly between the glasses.

6. Pour water in the baking dish.

7. Bake for 25 minutes.

8. Take out and serve.

9. Enjoy!

Nutrition (Per Serving)

Calories: 59

Fat: 2.4g

Carbohydrates: 7g

Protein: 3g

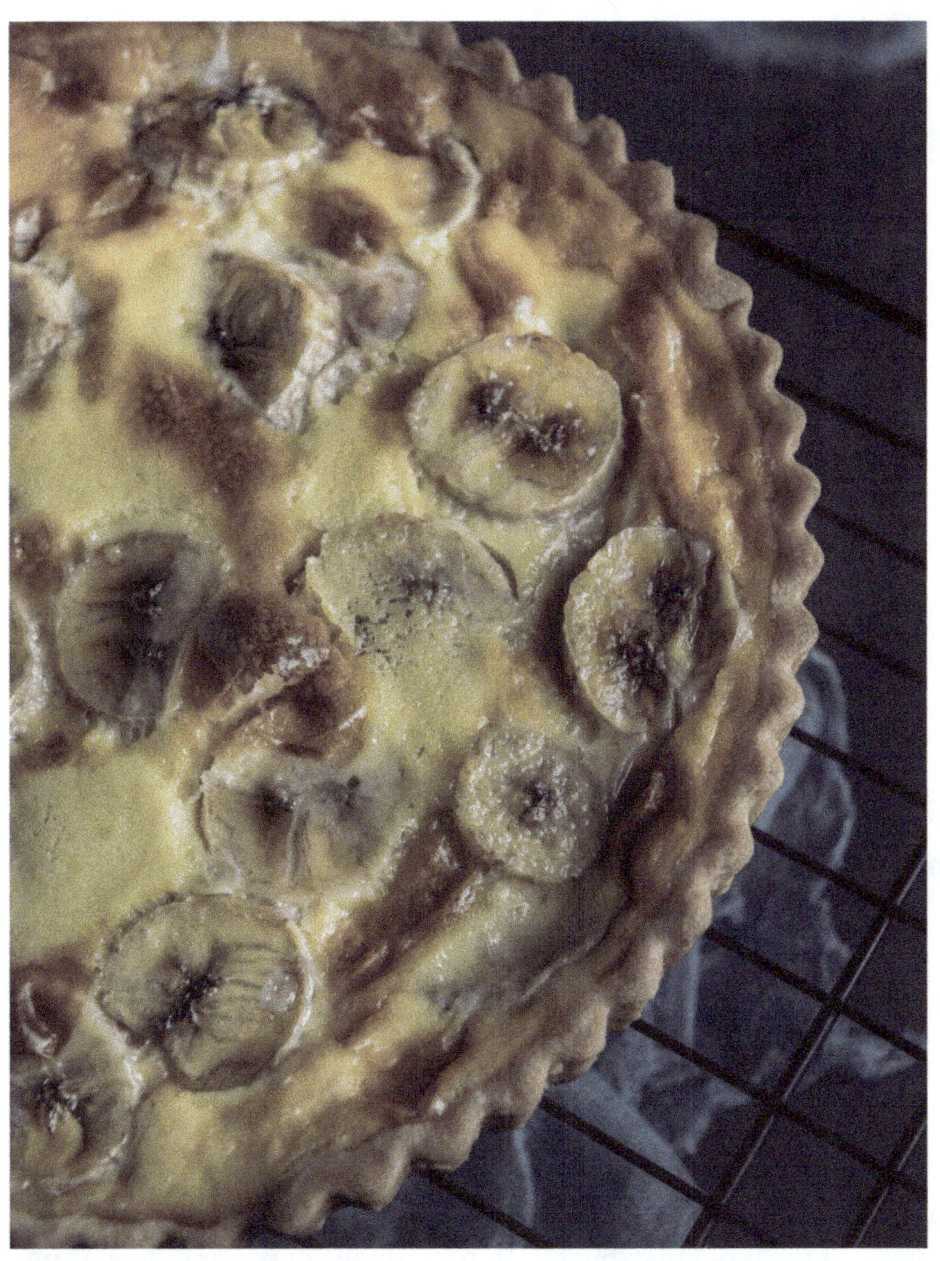

Healthy Tahini Buns

Serving: 3 buns

Prep Time: 10 minutes

Cooking Time: 15-20 minutes

Ingredients:

1 whole egg

5 tablespoons Tahini paste

½ teaspoon baking soda

1 teaspoon lemon juice

1 pinch salt

How To:

1. Pre-heat your oven to 350 degrees F.

2. Line a baking sheet with parchment paper and keep it on the side.

3. Add the listed ingredients to a blender and blend until you have a smooth batter.

4. Scoop batter onto prepared sheet forming buns.

5. Bake for 15-20 minutes.

6. Once done, remove from oven and let them cool.

7. Serve and enjoy!

Nutrition (Per Serving)

Total Carbs: 7g

Fiber: 2g

Protein: 6g

Fat: 14g

Calories: 172

Spicy Pecan Bowl

Serving: 3

Prep Time: 10 minutes

Cook Time: 120 minutes

Ingredients:

1-pound pecans, halved

2 tablespoons olive oil

1 teaspoon basil, dried

1 tablespoon chili powder

1 teaspoon oregano, dried

¼ teaspoon garlic powder

1 teaspoon rosemary, dried

½ teaspoon onion powder

How To:

1. Add pecans, oil, basil, chili powder, oregano, garlic powder, onion powder, rosemary and toss well.

2. Transfer to Slow Cooker and cook on LOW for 2 hours.

3. Divide between bowls and serve.

4. Enjoy!

Nutrition (Per Serving)

Calories: 152

Fat: 3g

Carbohydrates: 11g

Protein: 2g

Gentle Sweet Potato Tempura

Serving: 4

Prep Time: 15 minutes

Cook Time: 4 minutes

Ingredients:

2 whole eggs

½ teaspoon salt

3/4 cup ice water + 3 tablespoons ice water

¾ cup all-purpose flour + 1 tablespoons all-purpose flour 2 cups oil

1 sweet potato, scrubbed and sliced into 1/8-inch slices

For sauce

¼ cup rice wine

¼ cup coconut amines

How To:

1. Take a large bowl and beat in eggs until frothy.

2. Stir in salt, ice water, and flour, mix well until the batter is lumpy.

3. Take a frying pan and place over high heat, add oil and heat to 350 degrees F.

4. Dry-sweet potato slices and dip 3 slices at a time in the batter, let excess batter drip.

5. Fry until golden brown on both sides, each side should take about 2 minutes.

6. Live them out and drain excess oil, keep repeating until all potatoes are done.

7. Take a small bowl and whisk in rice wine, soy sauce and use it as a dipping sauce.

8. Enjoy!

Nutrition (Per Serving)

Calories: 315

Fat: 13g

Carbohydrates: 35g

Protein: 8g

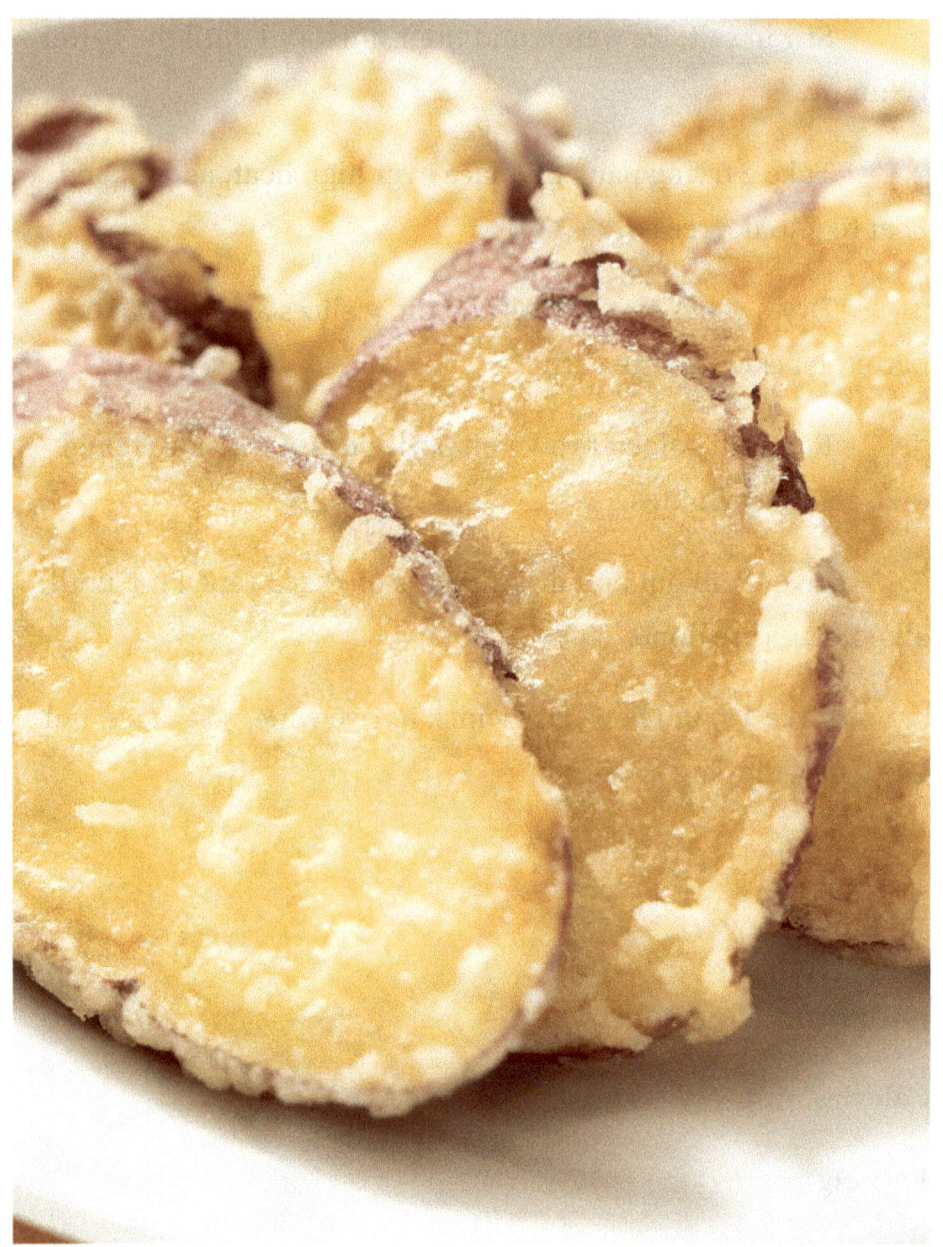

Japanese Cucumber Sunomono

Serving: 4

Prep Time: 15 minutes + 60 minutes chill time

Cook Time: Nil

Ingredients:

2 large sized cucumbers

1/3 cup of vinegar, rice

4 heaped teaspoons of sugar, white

1 heaped teaspoon of salt

1 ½ teaspoons freshly minced ginger root Seeds of sesame as needed

How To:

1. Cut cucumbers in half, lengthwise.
2. Scoop out any large seeds, slice crosswise into thin slices.

3. Take a small sized bowl and add ginger, salt, sugar and vinegar.

4. Mix thoroughly and add the cucumbers in the bowl.

5. Mix well to coat the cucumbers well.

6. Let it chill for about 1 hour.

7. Spread sesame and enjoy!

Nutrition (Per Serving)

Calories: 27

Fat: 0.2g

Carbohydrates: 6g

Protein: 0.6g

Radish and Hash Brown Dish

Serving: 4

Prep Time: 15 minutes + 60 minutes chill time

Cook Time: Nil

Ingredients:

1 pound radish, shredded

½ teaspoon onion powder

1/3 cup parmesan, grated

½ teaspoon garlic powder

4 whole eggs

Pepper to taste

How To:

1. Mix in radishes, pepper, onion, garlic powder, eggs, parmesan in bowl and stir well.

2. Arrange neatly on lined baking sheet.

3. Pre-heat your oven to 375 degrees F.

4. Transfer to oven and bake for 10 minutes.

5. Cut Hash Browns and enjoy!

Nutrition (Per Serving)

Calories: 60

Fat: 5g

Carbohydrates: 5g

Protein: 7g

Kid Friendly Popsicles

Serving: 4

Prep Time: 2 hours

Cook Time: 15 minutes

Ingredients:

1 ½ cups raspberries

2 cups water

How To:

1. Take a pan and add water and raspberries.

2. Heat over medium heat.

3. Bring the water to a boil and reduce heat.

4. Simmer for 15 minutes.

5. Remove from the heat and pour mix into ice cube tray.

6. Add popsicle stick in each and chill for 2 hours.

7. Serve and enjoy!

Nutrition (Per Serving)

Calories: 58

Fat: 0.4g

Carbohydrates: 0g

Protein: 1.4g

The Pear and Chocolate Catastrophe

Serving: 2

Prep Time: 5 minutes

Ingredients:

1 banana (freckled skin)

2-3 pears

2 tablespoons hulled hemp seeds

1 bag frozen raspberries

2 ½ cups coconut water

1 teaspoon raw chocolate

Small bunch arugula lettuce leaves

Liquid stevia

How To:

1. Add all the listed ingredients to your blender.

2. Blend until smooth.

3. Add a few ice cubes and serve the smoothie.

4. Enjoy!

Nutrition (Per Serving)

Calories: 200

Fat: 10g

Carbohydrates: 14g

Protein 2g

The Avocado Paradise

Serving: 2

Prep Time: 5 minutes

Ingredients:

½ avocado, cubed

1 cup coconut milk

Half a lemon

¼ cup fresh spinach leaves

1 pear

1 tablespoon hemp seed powder

Toppings:

Handful of macadamia nuts

Handful of grapes

2 lemon slices

How To:

1. Blend all the ingredients until smooth.

2. Add a few ice cubes to make it chilled.

3. Add your desired toppings.

4. Enjoy!

Nutrition (Per Serving)

Calories: 200

Fat: 10g

Carbohydrates: 14g

Protein 2g

The Authentic Vegetable Medley

Serving: 2

Prep Time: 5 minutes

Ingredients:

1 cup broccoli, steamed

1 bunch asparagus, steamed

2 cups coconut milk

2 tablespoons coconut oil

2 carrots, peeled

Few inches of horseradish

Himalayan salt

Pinch of chili powder

½ onion

2 garlic cloves

How To:

1. Add all the listed ingredients to your blender except coconut oil, salt and chili powder.

2. Blend until smooth.

3. Add salt, coconut oil and chili powder.

4. Stir well and serve chilled!

Nutrition (Per Serving)

Calories: 200

Fat: 10g

Carbohydrates: 14g

Protein 2g

The Original Power Producer

Serving: 2

Prep Time: 5 minutes

Ingredients:

½ cup spinach

1 avocado, diced

1 cup coconut milk

1 tablespoon flaxseed

2 nori sheets, roasted and crushed

1 garlic clove Salt to taste

Toppings:

Handful of pistachios

3 tablespoons bell pepper, finely chopped

Handful of parsley leaves

How To:

1. Blend all the ingredients until smooth.

2. Add a few ice cubes to make it chilled.

3. Add your desired toppings.

4. Enjoy!

Nutrition (Per Serving)

Calories: 200

Fat: 10g

Carbohydrates: 14g

Protein 2g

The Dreamy Cherry Mix

Serving: 2

Prep Time: 5 minutes

Ingredients:

½ cup ripe cherries

Juice of 1 lemon

1 cup coconut milk

1 avocado, cubed

¼ cup spinach

Few slices of cucumber, peeled

Toppings:

Handful of pistachios

Handful of raisins

1 slice lemon

How To:

1. Blend all the ingredients until smooth.

2. Add a few ice cubes to make it chilled.

3. Add your desired toppings.

4. Enjoy!

Nutrition (Per Serving)

Calories: 200

Fat: 10g

Carbohydrates: 14g

Protein 2g

Lemon Smoothie

Serving: 2

Prep Time: 5 minutes

Ingredients:

2 cups organic rice milk, gluten free

1 cup melon, chopped

½ avocado, cubed

½ cucumber, peeled and sliced

Ice cubes

2 limes, juiced

1 tablespoon coconut oil

Few banana slices to taste

How To:

1. Add the listed ingredients to your blender (except

coconut oil) and blend well.

2. Blend until you have a smooth texture.

3. Add coconut oil and stir.

4. Enjoy!

Nutrition (Per Serving)

Calories: 200

Fat: 10g

Carbohydrates: 14g

Protein 2g

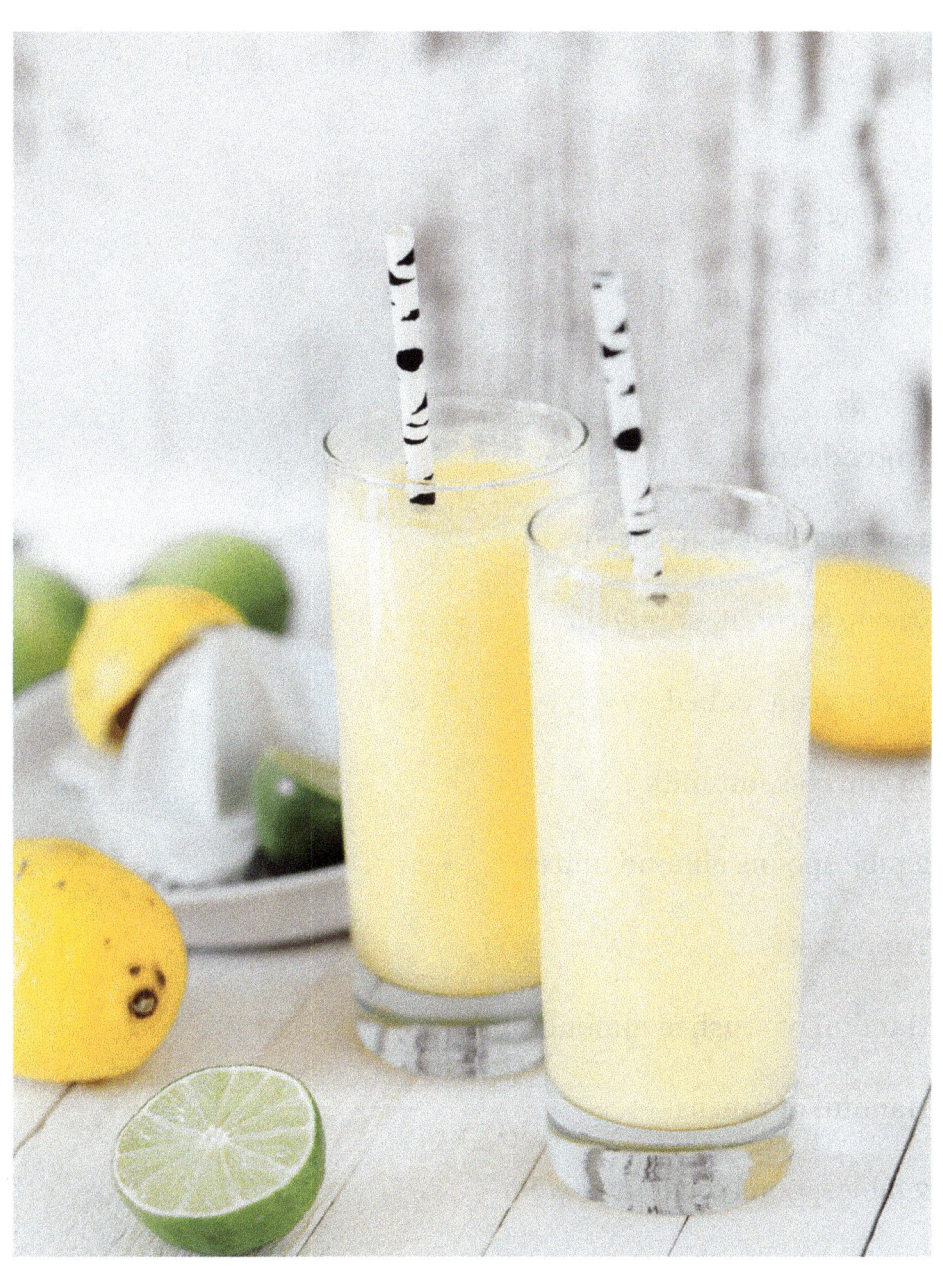

One The Watermelon

Serving: 2

Prep Time: 5 minutes

Ingredients:

1 cup watermelon, sliced

½ cup coconut, shredded

1 grapefruit, cubed

½ cup coconut milk

2 tablespoons almond butter

Toppings:

Handful of crushed almonds

Handful of raisins

2 tablespoons coconut powder

How To:

1. Blend all the ingredients until smooth.

2. Add a few ice cubes to make it chilled.

3. Add your desired toppings.

4. Enjoy!

Nutrition (Per Serving)

Calories: 200

Fat: 10g

Carbohydrates: 14g

Protein 2g

Strawberry and Rhubarb Smoothie

Serving: 1

Prep Time: 5 minutes

Cook Time: 3 minutes

Ingredients:

1 rhubarb stalk, chopped

1 cup fresh strawberries, sliced

½ cup plain Greek yoghurt

Pinch of ground cinnamon

3 ice cubes

How To:

1. Take a small saucepan and fill with water over high heat.
2. Bring to boil and add rhubarb, boil for 3 minutes.

3. Drain and transfer to a blender.

4. Add strawberries, honey, yogurt, cinnamon and pulse mixture until smooth.

5. Add ice cubes and blend until thick and has no lumps.

6. Pour into glass and enjoy chilled.

Nutrition (Per Serving)

Calories: 295

Fat: 8g

Carbohydrates: 56g

Protein: 6g

Decisive Cauliflower and Mushroom Risotto

Serving: 4

Prep Time: 10 minutes

Cook Time: 20 minutes

Ingredients:

1 cup vegetable stock

head cauliflower, grated

9 ounces mushroom, chopped

tablespoons almond butter

Sunflower seeds and black pepper, to taste 1 cup coconut cream

How To:

1. Take a saucepan and pour stock into it.
2. Bring it to boil and set it aside.

3. Then take a skillet and melt almond butter over medium heat.

4. Add mushroom to sauté until it turns golden brown.

5. Stir in stock and grated cauliflower.

6. Bring the mixture to a simmer and add cream.

7. Cook until liquid is reduced and cauliflower is al dente.

8. Serve warm and enjoy!

Nutrition (Per Serving)

Calories: 186

Fat: 16.5g

Carbohydrates: 6.7g

Protein: 2.8g

Authentic Zucchini Boats

Serving: 4

Prep Time: 10 minutes

Cook Time: 25 minutes

Ingredients:

4 medium zucchini

½ cup marinara sauce

¼ red onion, sliced

¼ cup kalamata olives, chopped

½ cup cherry tomatoes, sliced

2 tablespoons fresh basil

How To:

1. Pre-heat your oven to 400 degrees F.
2. Cut the zucchini half-lengthwise and shape them in boats.

3. Take a bowl and add tomato sauce, spread 1 layer of sauce on top of each of the boat.

4. Top with onion, olives, and tomatoes.

5. Bake for 20-25 minutes.

6. Top with basil and enjoy!

Nutrition (Per Serving)

Calories: 278

Fat: 20g

Carbohydrates: 10g

Protein: 15g

Roasted Onions and Green Beans

Serving: 6

Prep Time: 10 minutes

Cook Time: 15 minutes

Ingredients:

1 yellow onion, sliced into rings

½ teaspoon onion powder

2 tablespoons coconut flour

1 1/3 pounds fresh green beans, trimmed and chopped

How To:

1. Take a large bowl and mix sunflower seeds with onion powder and coconut flour.

2. Add onion rings.

3. Mix well to coat.

4. Spread the rings in the baking sheet, lined with parchment paper.

5. Drizzle with some oil.

6. Bake for 10 minutes at 400 degrees F.

7. Parboil the green beans for 3 to 5 minutes in the boiling water.

8. Drain and serve the beans with baked onion rings.

9. Serve warm and enjoy!

Nutrition (Per Serving)

Calories: 214

Fat: 19.4g

Carbohydrates:3.7g

Protein: 8.3g

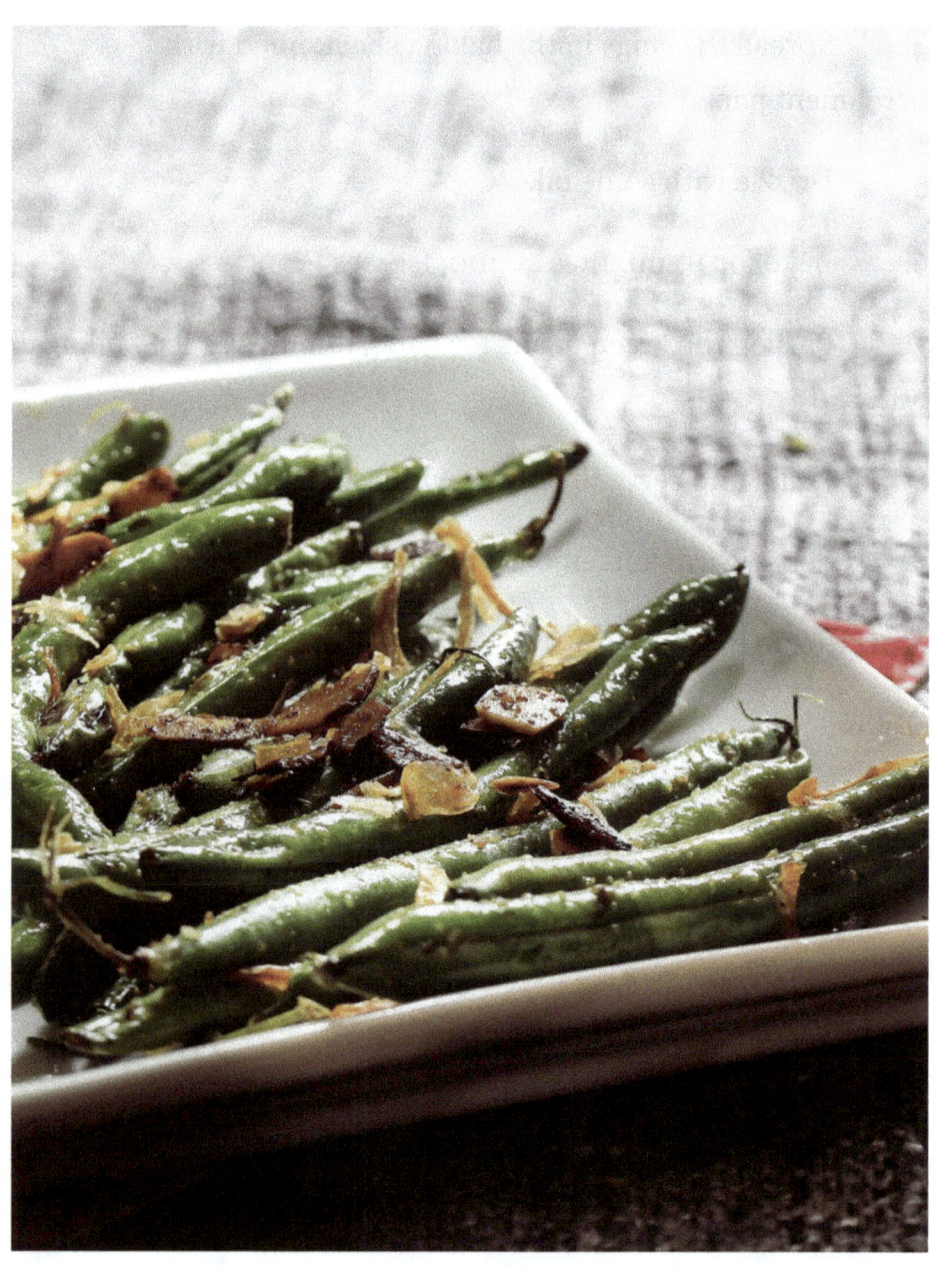

Sugar Break Apple and Peanut Butter Oatmeal

Ingredients

1 cup steel-cut oats

Three medium-large Granny Smith apples, cored and sliced into 1-2" chunks

A swirl of peanut butter

pinch ground cinnamon

1 tbsp butter (optional)

4 cups of water

pinch salt

Directions

Cook the oats till they reach the specified texture and creaminess.

Cut apples, toss them into the oats, and stir.

Then add spread into it and stir until melted and spread throughout.

Top with a touch of cinnamon and butter (optional) and enjoy!

Nutrient Calories: 453

Sweet Potato Toast

Ingredients

One potato (sweet)

Instructions

1. Divide the sweet potato into 1/4-inch slices and pop into the toaster.

2. Top with anything you select. Popular combinations include spread with fruit, avocado, hummus, eggs, cheese, and tuna fish salad.

Nutrient Calories: 112

Granelli

Ingredients

4 cups rolled oats

2 cups raw cashews

2 cups raw walnuts

2 cups of raw almonds

2 cups of fresh sunflower seed

2 cups of raw pumpkin seeds

3 cups unsweetened coconut flakes

1/2 cup of maple liquid syrup

1/4 cup of unrefined coconut oil, plus 2 tsp for oiling the baking sheet

pinch of sea salt

1/3 cup of pure orange oil

2 cups of organic raisins

2 cups of dried cherries or cranberries

Directions

1. Set the oven to 300°F.

2. during a considerable bowl, mix the oats, nuts, seeds, and coconut flakes.

3. Take a little bowl, stir together the syrup, copra oil, salt, and orange oil till well combined, then pour over the oat-nut combination and blend nicely.

4. Spread granola on an outsized oiled baking sheet (do it in batches if needed) and bake for 35-forty minutes until golden brown (rotate the baking sheet halfway via for even baking).

5. Remove from oven and permit refreshing absolutely before mixing with raisins and dried cherries or cranberries.

6. Store in airtight place within the fridge to stay extra crispiness.

Tofu Turmeric Scramble

Ingredients

One 8-ounce block of firm or extra-firm tofu, drained 1 tbsp extra virgin olive oil ¼ red onion, chopped

One green or purple bell pepper, chopped 2 cups of clean spinach, loosely chopped ½ cup sliced button mushrooms ½ tsp every salt and pepper

1 tsp garlic powder

½ tbsp turmeric

¼ cup nutritional yeast

Directions

1. Drain the tofu and squeeze lightly to try to to away with extra water. Crumble tofu right into a bowl with the help of hand - the smaller the pieces, the higher.

2. Prep vegetables and region an outsized skillet at medium temperature. Once ready, then add vegetable oil, onions, and bell peppers. Mix during a pinch of the salt and pepper and

prepare dinner for about five minutes to melt the vegetables. Then add mushrooms and sauté for two mins. Then upload tofu. Sauté for about three minutes, a touch more if the tofu is watery.

3. Add the remainder of the salt, pepper, garlic turmeric, and nutritional yeast and blend with a spatula, ensuring the spices combo well. Cook for an additional 5 to eight mins till tofu is lightly browned.

4. Add the spinach and canopy the pan so as to steam for 2 minutes. Serve immediately with facets of your choice.

Nutrient Calories: 158

Whole Grain Cheese Pancakes

Ingredients

1 cup of oat flour

1/2 cup of sorghum flour

2 tbsp of teff flour

1/3 cup of plus 1 tbsp, tapioca starch

1 tbsp of baking powder

1/2 of tsp salt

3 1/2 of tsp sugar

1/2 tsp of flax meal

3/4 cup of buttermilk

1/3 cup of cottage cheese

Three eggs

half tsp vanilla extract

4 tsp canola oil

1-pint blueberries

1/2 cup maple syrup

3 tbsp water

1 tsp lemon juice

pinch of salt

Instructions

1.   Combine all of your dry elements during a huge bowl and stir to combine evenly.

2.   Whisk all of your wet ingredients in another bowl collectively.

3.   Make a hole within the center of your dry substances and start to slowly pour within the wet materials, a few quarter cup at a time. this may confirm that no lumps form when whisking.

4.   Continue including your wet components to the flour base till a smooth batter form. Let the batter relax for quarter-hour at an equivalent time as you preheat your grill.

5.   While the grill is warming up, make a warm maple blueberry compote. Mix blueberries, syrup, water, lemon juice, and a pinch salt during a small pot. Stir frivolously to combine.

6. Gently heat the pot over medium-low warmth till the blueberries start to pop and release their natural juices. Set aside, but maintain heat.

7. Once the grill is preheated to a medium-hot temperature, lightly oil the restaurant employing a nonstick spray or a small amount of neutral-flavored oil.

8. Ladle the batter on to the skillet, ensuring you are doing not overload it.

9. Give time to the pancakes to cook undisturbed until the looks of the sides dry and bubbles come to the surface without breaking. This has got to take roughly minutes.

10. Flip the pancakes over and cook at the opposite facet for an additional two minutes.

11. Keep heat or serve immediately with the sweet and comfy maple-blueberry compote.

Nutrient Calories: 511

Red Pepper, Kale, and Cheddar Frittata

Ingredients

1 tsp olive oil

5 oz baby kale and spinach

One red pepper, diced

1/3 cup sliced scallions

12 eggs

3/4 cup milk

1 cup sharp shredded cheddar cheese

1/4 tsp salt

1/4 tsp pepper

Directions

1. Preheat oven to 375 ☐.

2. Spray an eight 1/2-inch by using 12-inch glass or casserole dish with vegetable oil or nonstick spray.

3. Heat oil during a large frypan. Add crimson peppers on low and cook until tender. Add kale and spinach, on occasion stirring till vegetables are wilted, or for about three min.

4. Transfer peppers and greens to the plate, spreading evenly. Add sliced scallions.

5. Beat eggs with milk, salt, and pepper. Pour the egg aggregate over the pan. Sprinkle cheese on top.

6. Bake about 35-40 mins or till the mixture is totally set and starting to lightly brown. For extra color, place under broiler for an extra 1 to 3 minutes, watching to make sure the highest doesn't burn. Let cool about five mins before cutting it.

7. Serve it as warm or refrigerate for a fast breakfast during the week

— microwave for 1-2 minutes to reheat.

Nutrient Calories: 77

Scrambled Eggs with Bell Pepper and Feta

Ingredients

Olive oil-Salad or cooking-1 tsp-4.5 grams

Green bell pepper-Sweet, green, raw-2 medium (approx 2-3/4" long, 2-1/2" dia)-238 grams Egg-Whole, fresh eggs-Four large-200 grams Feta cheese-1 oz-28.4 grams

Directions

1. Heat the oil during a skillet on medium heat. Add chopped peppers and cook till tender.

2. Stir the eggs and increase the skillet with the peppers. Stir slowly over medium-low heat till they attain your preferred doneness. Sprinkle inside the feta cheese and stir to combine and soften the cheese. Serve directly and luxuriate in it!

Nutrient

Calories 448 Carbs 14g Fat 30g Protein 31g Fiber 4g Net carbs 10g Sodium 551mg Cholesterol 769mg

Devilled Egg Toast

Ingredients

Egg-Whole, fresh eggs-Two large-100 grams Mustard-Prepared, yellow-2 tbsp-30 grams

Light mayonnaise-Salad dressing, Kraft brand-2 tbsp-30 grams Whole-wheat bread-Commercially prepared-Four slice-112 grams

Directions

1. Place egg during a bowl and canopy with water. Boil the water, remove from heat, cover, and let sit 10 minutes. Drain under cold water, peel, and mash.

2. Combine egg with the mustard and mayonnaise. Mix well.

3. Toast bread and top with egg mixture. Enjoy!

Nutrition

Calories 543 Carbs 53g Fat 24g Protein 28g Fiber 8g Net carbs 45g Sodium 1173mg Cholesterol 382mg

Basic Scrambled Eggs

Ingredients

Egg-Whole, fresh eggs-Six large-300 grams

Butter-Unsalted-1 tbsp-14.2 grams

Chives-Raw-1 tbsp chopped-3 grams

Tarragon-Spices, dried-1 tbsp, ground-4.8 grams

Table-One dash-0.40 grams

Pepper-Spices, black-One dash-0.10 grams

Directions

1.   Beat the eggs during a bowl and till damaged up. Sprinkle with a pinch each of salt and pepper and beat to include. Place tablespoons of the eggs during a small bowl; put aside.

2.   Heat a 10-inch nonstick frypan over medium-low warmth until hot, approximately 2 minutes. Add butter to the pan and therefore the usage of a rubber spatula, swirl until it's melted and foamy, and therefore the box is flippantly coated. Pour within the massive a part of the eggs, sprinkle with chives and

tarragon (if the usage of), and let sit down undisturbed till eggs just start to line round the edges, about 1 to 2 minutes. Using the rubber spatula, push the eggs from the edges into the center. After30 seconds repeat pushing the eggs from the sides into the middle every 30 seconds till simply set, for a complete cooking time of about 5 minutes.

3. Add the last word tablespoons raw egg and stir till eggs not look wet. Remove from warmness and season with salt and pepper as required. Serve immediately.

Nutrition

Calories 546 Carbs 5g Fat 40g Protein 39g Fiber 0g Net carbs 4g Sodium 586mg Cholesterol 1147mg

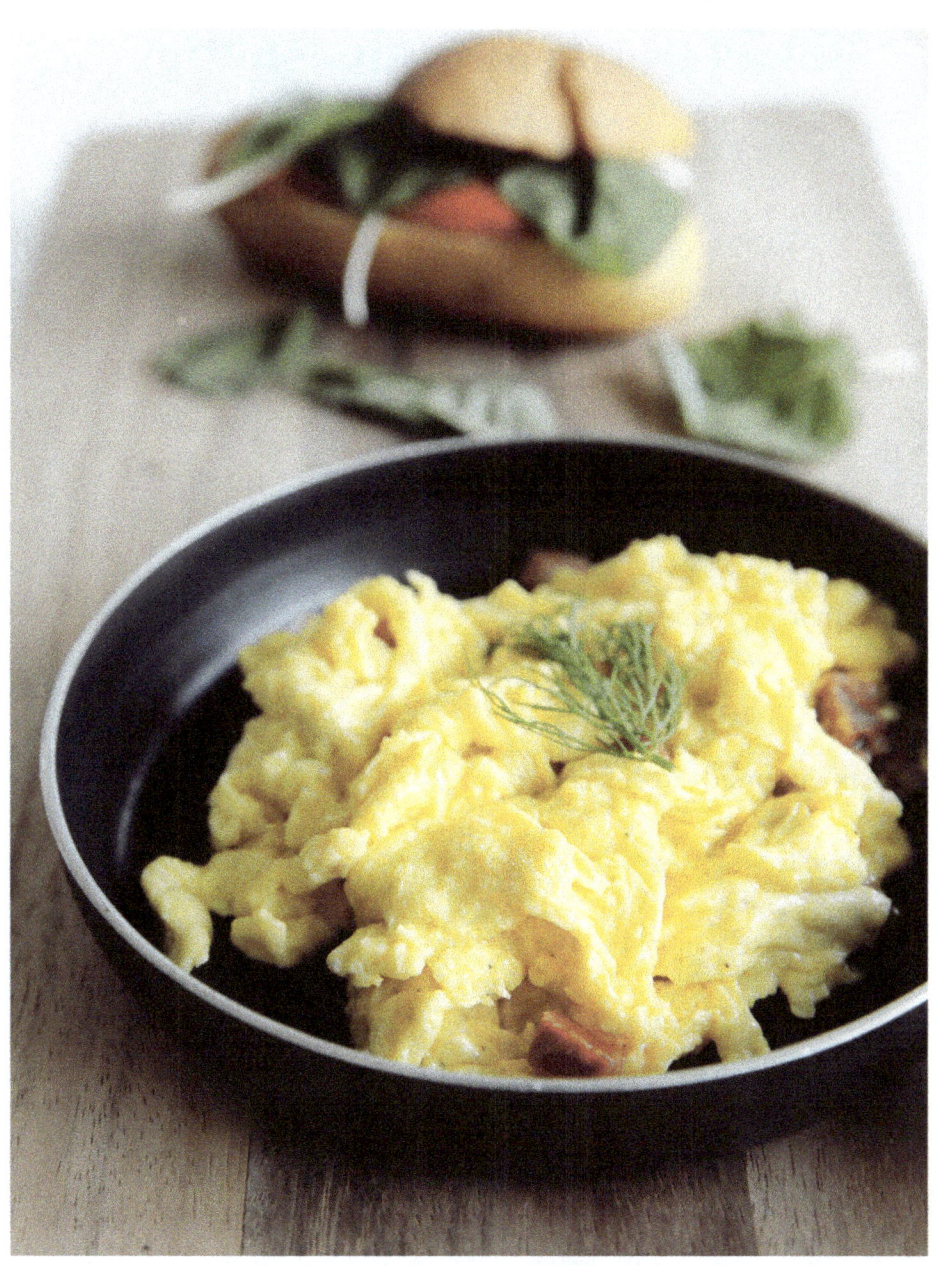

Baked Butternut-Squash Rigatoni

Ingredients

One large butternut squash

Three clove garlic

2 tbsp. olive oil

1 lb. rigatoni

1/2 c. heavy cream

3 c. shredded fontina

2 tbsp. chopped fresh sage

1 tbsp. salt

1 tsp. freshly ground pepper

1 c. panko breadcrumbs

Directions

1. Set oven at 425 degrees. At an equivalent time, take an outsized bowl and toss garlic, squash, and vegetable oil for

coating. Take a baking sheet and roast for about hour. Then calm for 20 minutes. Reduce oven to 350 degrees.

2.	Then, boil the salted water and cook rigatoni consistent with package directions. Drain and put aside .

3.	employing a blender, purée reserved squash with cream until smooth.

4.	Take an outsized bowl and blend squash puree with reserved rigatoni, 2 cups fontina, sage, salt, and pepper. Apply olive oil on the edges of the baking pan. Transfer rigatoni-squash mixture to plate.

5.	Take a little bowl, combine the remaining fontina and panko. Sprinkle over pasta and bake until golden brown,20 to 25 minutes.

Simple Caprese Sandwich

Ingredients

Sourdough bread, French or Vienna, Two slices, 192 grams Mozzarella cheese

Whole milk 2 oz 56.7 grams

Tomatoes - Red, ripe, raw, year-round average

Four slices, medium (1/4" thick)

Instructions

Cut a large slice of sourdough in half (or use two small slices). Top one slice with 1oz of sliced mozzarella and then two slices of tomatoes. The flavor is mild, so season with salt pepper if desired.

Nutrition

Calories707 Carbs104g Fat17g Protein34g Fiber5g Net carbs99g Sodium1515mg Cholesterol45mg

Cottage Cheese Honey Toast

Ingredients

Whole-wheat bread-Commercially prepared-Two slice-56 grams

Cottage cheese- 1% milkfat-1 cup, (not packed)-226 grams

Honey-2 tbsp-42 grams

Directions

Toast bread to your liking. Spread with cottage cheese and drizzle with honey. Enjoy!

Nutrition

Calories432 Carbs65g Fat4g Protein35g Fiber3g Net carbs61g Sodium1174mg Cholesterol9mg

Pimento Cheese Sandwich

Ingredients

Pimento cheese-Pasteurized process-2 oz-56.7 grams Multi-grain bread-Four slices regular-104 grams

Directions

1. Spread the pimento cheese on each side of bread. And then on the other slice of bread to form a sandwich. Enjoy!

Nutrition

Calories488 Carbs46g Fat22g Protein26g Fiber8g Net carbs38g Sodium915mg Cholesterol53mg

Tomato Salad

Ingredients

Vinegar-Cider-2 2/3 tbsp-39.4 grams

Cucumber-Peeled, raw-Two medium-402 grams

Onions-Raw-1/2 large-75 grams

Tomatoes-Red, ripe, fresh, year-round average

Three medium whole (2-3/5" dia)-369 grams

Water-Plain, clean water-1/2 cup-118 grams

Directions

Peel and slice cucumbers into coins. Cut tomatoes into pieces. Dice red onion. Add vinegar and water and mix well.

Nutrition

Calories153 Carbs31g Fat1g Protein6g Fiber9g Net carbs22g Sodium32mg Cholesterol0mg

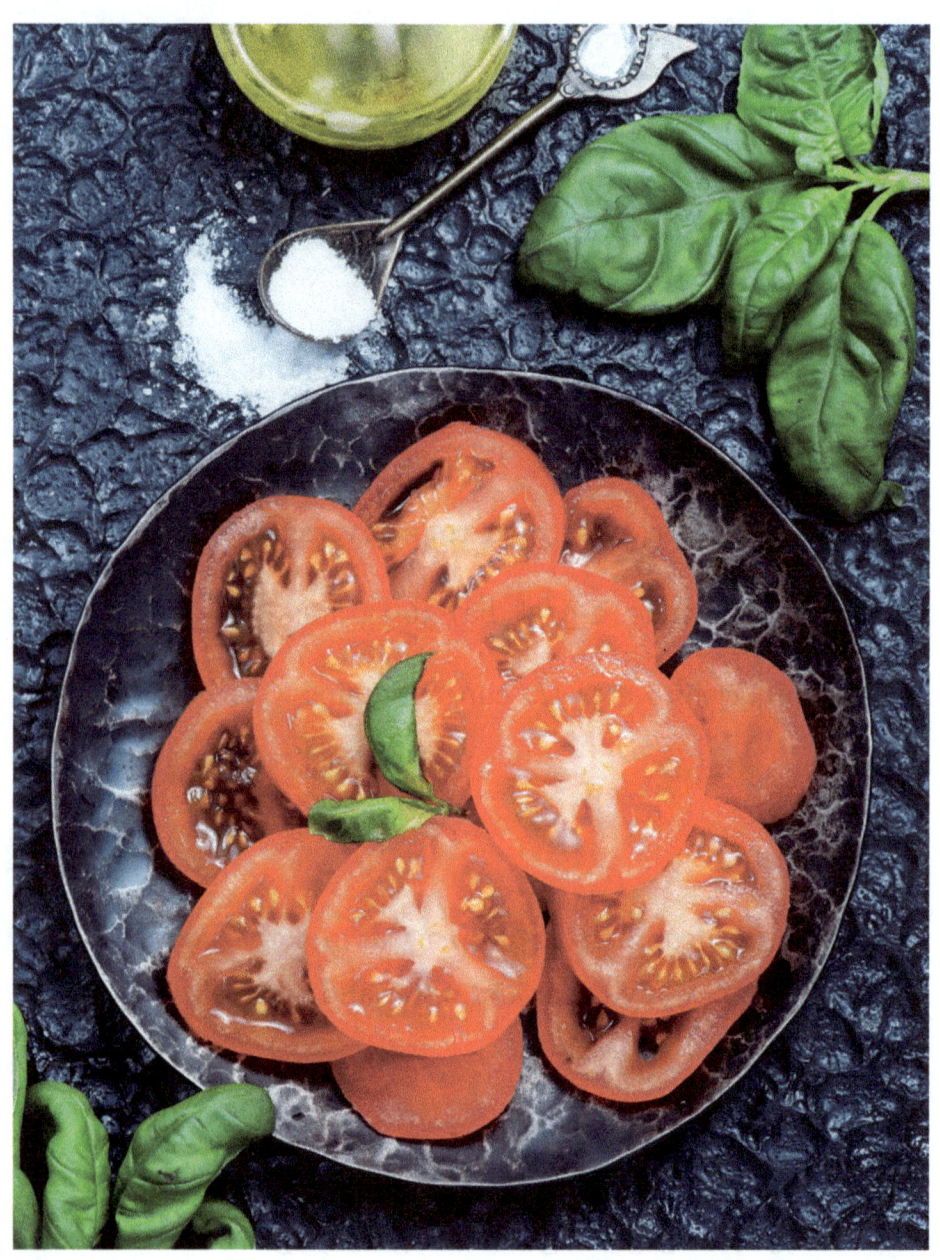

Tomato and Cheese Wrap

Ingredients

Tortillas-2 tortilla -92 grams

mayonnaise-like dressing-Regular, with salt-2 tbsp-29.4 grams

Tomatoes-Two medium whole -246 grams

Lettuce-2 cup shredded-144 grams

Cheddar cheese-2 oz-56.7 grams

Directions

1. Lightly spread mayo on tortilla shell.

2. Cut tomatoes however you like them.

3. Layer ingredients, spreading them over the tortilla.

4. Tuck up about an inch the side of the shell you've decided is the bottom and roll up the wrap. Enjoy!

Nutrition

Calories638 Carbs66g Fat32g Protein25g Fiber7g Net carbs59g Sodium1236mg Cholesterol63mg

Peanut Butter Yogurt

Ingredients

Nonfat greek yogurt-1 cup-240 grams

Peanut butter-2 tbsp-32 grams

Vanilla extract-1 tsp-2.2 grams

Directions

Combine ingredients and enjoy it!

Nutrition

Calories345 Carbs16g Fat17g Protein32g Fiber2g Net carbs15g Sodium223mg Cholesterol12mg

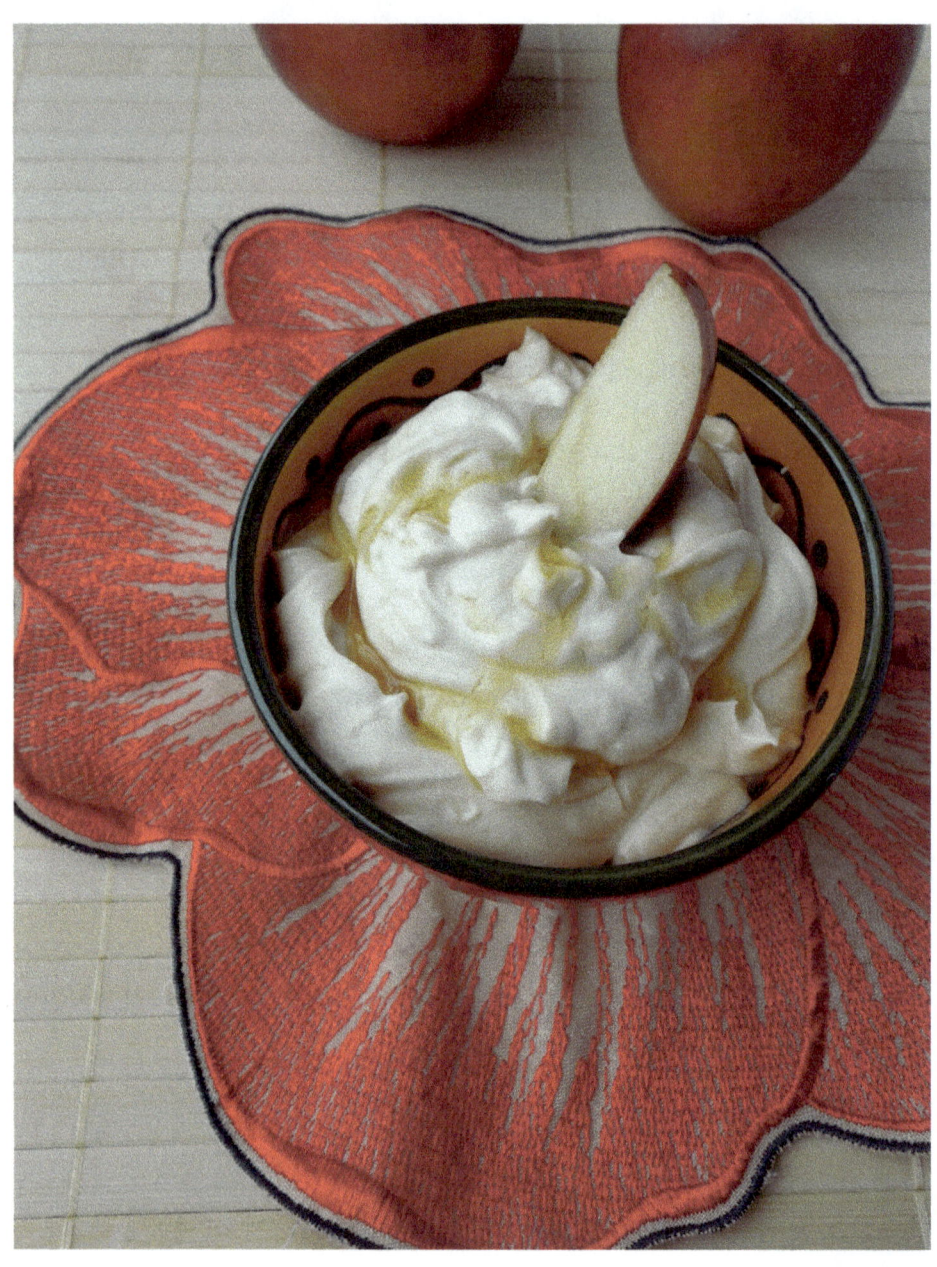

Peanut Butter & Carrots

Ingredients

Peanut butter-4 tbsp-64 grams

Carrots-2 cup chopped-256 grams

Directions

Spread peanut butter on carrots and enjoy!

Nutrition

Calories482 Carbs38g Fat33g Protein18g Fiber12g Net carbs26g Sodium188mg Cholesterol0mg

Cucumber Tomato Salad with Tuna

Ingredients

Tomatoes-Two medium whole -246 grams

Lettuce-1 cup shredded-36 grams

Cucumber-With peel, raw-One cucumber-301 grams

Tuna-One can-165 grams

Directions

1. Chop vegetables and lettuce.
2. Toss together with the tuna and enjoy it!

Nutrition

Calories237 Carbs22g Fat2g Protein37g Fiber5g Net carbs17g Sodium436mg Cholesterol59mg

Peanut butter and Jelly

Ingredients

Multi-grain bread-Four slices regular-104 grams

Butter-Unsalted-2 tsp-9.5 grams

Peanut butter-Smooth style, without salt-3 tbsp-48 grams

Jams and preserves-2 tbsp-40 grams

Directions

1. Toast the bread, and it's optionally. Drizzle 1/2 teaspoon of butter on all sides of the bread.

2. Spread butter on one side and jam on another side.

Nutrition

Calories 742 Carbs 83g Fat 37g Protein 25g Fiber 11g Net carbs 73g Sodium 418mg Cholesterol 20mg

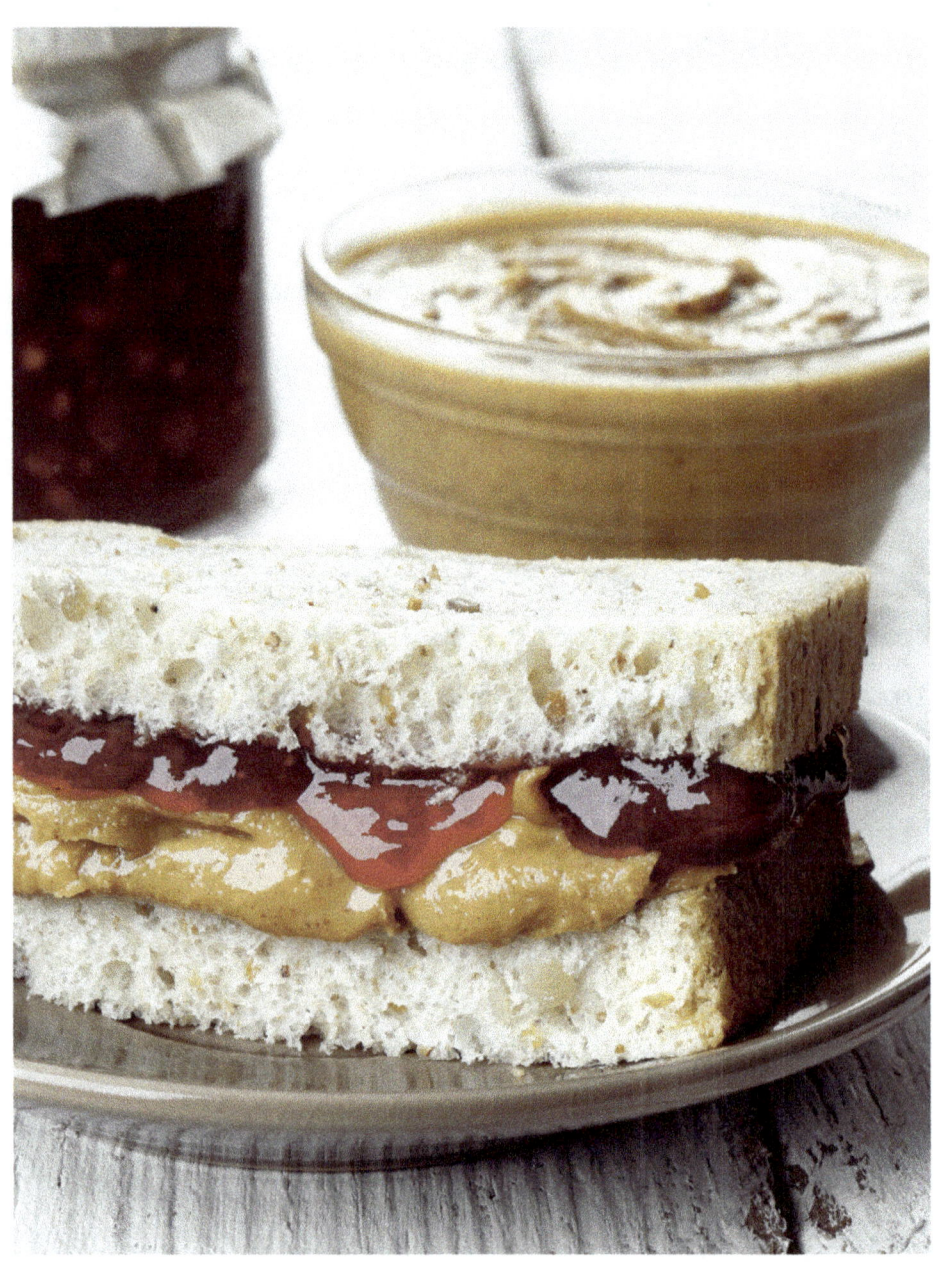

Chicken Scampi Pasta

Ingredients

1 pound of thinly-sliced chicken cutlets, cut into 1/2-inch-thick strips

Three tablespoons olive oil

Eight tablespoons unsalted butter, cubed Six cloves garlic, sliced

1/2 teaspoon crushed red pepper flakes

1/2 cup dry white wine

12 ounces angel hair pasta

One teaspoon lemon zest plus the juice of 1 large lemon 1/2 cup freshly grated Parmesan

1/2 cup chopped fresh Italian parsley

Directions

1.   Take a huge pot of salted water to a boil for the pasta. Sprinkle the chook with a couple of salts. Heat a huge skillet over medium-high warmth until hot, then upload the oil.

Working in 2 batches, brown the chook until golden however not cooked through, 2 to a couple of minutes keep with batch. Remove the chicken to a plate.

2.	Melt four tablespoons of the butter within the skillet. Add the garlic and crimson pepper flakes and cook dinner until the garlic begins to show golden at the sides, 30 seconds to 1 minute. Add the wine, deliver to a simmer, and cook dinner till reduced by using half, approximately 2 minutes. Remove from the heat.

3.	Meanwhile, cook dinner the pasta till very hard, reserving 1 cup of the pasta water. Add the pasta and 3/four cup pasta water to the skillet alongside the hen, lemon peel and juice, and therefore the last four tablespoons butter. Return the skillet to medium-low warmness and gently stir the pasta until the butter is melted, including the last word 1/four pasta water if the pasta appears too dry. Remove the skillet from the heat, sprinkle with the cheese and parsley and toss before serving.

Apple-Cherry Pork Medallions

Ingredients

One pork tenderloin (1 pound)

One teaspoon minced fresh rosemary or 1/4 teaspoon dried rosemary, crushed

One teaspoon minced fresh thyme or 1/4 teaspoon dried thyme

1/2 teaspoon celery salt

One tablespoon olive oil

One large apple, sliced

2/3 cup unsweetened apple juice

Three tablespoons dried tart cherries

One tablespoon honey

One tablespoon cider vinegar

One package (8.8 ounces) ready-to-serve brown rice

Instructions

1. Cut tenderloin crosswise into 12 slices; sprinkle with rosemary, thyme and flavorer. during a huge skillet, heat oil over medium-excessive heat. Brown pork on both sides; do away with from pan.

2. In the equal skillet, combine apple, fruit juice, cherries, honey and vinegar. Boil it and stirring to loosen browned bits from pan. Reduce warmness; simmer, uncovered, 3-four minutes or simply till apple is tender.

3. Return meat to the pan, turning to coat with sauce; cook, covered, 3-4 minutes or till meat is tender. Meanwhile, put together rice keep with package deal directions; serve with meat mixture.

Nutrition Facts

349 calories, 9g fat (2g saturated fat), 64mg cholesterol, 179mg sodium, 37g carbohydrate (16g sugars, 4g fibre), and 25g protein.

Butternut Turkey Soup

Ingredients

Three shallots, thinly sliced

One tsp of olive oil

3 cups of reduced-sodium chicken broth

3 cups of cubed peeled butternut squash (3/4-inch cubes) Two medium-sized red potatoes, cut into 1/2-inch cubes 1-1/2 cups of water

Two teaspoons of minced fresh thyme

1/2 teaspoon pepper

Two whole cloves

3 cups cubed cooked turkey breast

Instructions

1. In a large-size saucepan coated with cooking spray, cook dinner shallots in oil over medium heat till tender. Stir within the broth, squash, potatoes, water, thyme and pepper.

2.   Place spices on a double thickness of cheesecloth; carry up corners of the material and tie with string to shape a bag. Stir into soup. bring back a boil. Reduce warmness; cowl and simmer for 10-15 mins or till vegetables are tender. Stir in turkey; warmth through. Discard spice bag.

Nutrition

192 calories, 2g fat (0 saturated fat), 60mg cholesterol, 332mg sodium, 20g carbohydrate (3g sugars, 3g fibre), 25g protein.

Black Bean & Sweet Potato Rice Bowls

Ingredients

3/4 cup uncooked long-grain rice

1/4 teaspoon garlic salt

1-1/2 cups water

Three tablespoons olive oil, divided

One large sweet potato, peeled and diced

One medium red onion, finely chopped

4 cups chopped fresh kale (sturdy stems removed) One can (15 ounces) black beans, rinsed and drained Two tablespoons sweet chilli sauce Lime wedges, optional

Additional sweet chilli sauce, optional

Instructions

1. Place rice, flavorer and water during a large saucepan; bring back a boil. Reduce heat; simmer, covered until liquid is

absorbed and rice is tender 15-20 minutes. Remove from heat; let stand 5 minutes.

2.   At an equivalent time take an outsized pan and warmth two tablespoons oil over medium-high heat; saute sweet potato 8 minutes. Add onion; cook and stir until potato is tender 4-6 minutes. Add kale; cook and stir until tender, 3-5 minutes. Stir in beans; heat through.

3.   Gently stir two tablespoons chilli sauce and remaining oil into rice; increase potato mixture. If you would like , serve with lime wedges and extra chilli sauce.

Nutrition

435 calories, 11g fat (2g saturated fat), 0 cholesterol, 405mg sodium, 74g carbohydrate (15g sugars, 8g fibre), 10g protein.

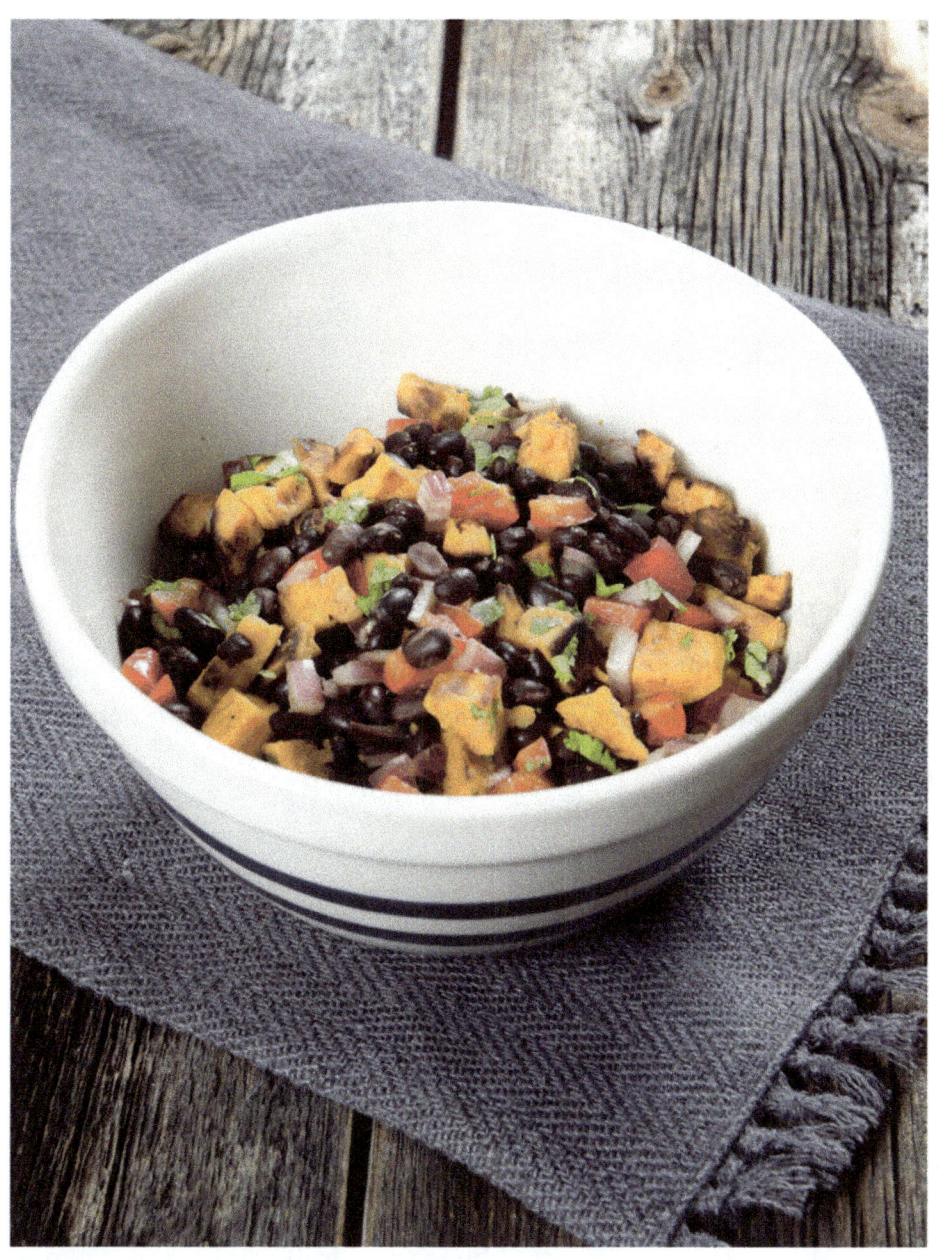

Pepper Ricotta Primavera

Ingredients

1 cup part-skim ricotta cheese

1/2 cup fat-free milk

Four teaspoons olive oil

One garlic clove, minced

1/2 teaspoon crushed red pepper flakes One medium green pepper, julienned One medium sweet red pepper, julienned One medium fresh yellow pepper, julienned One medium zucchini, sliced 1 cup frozen peas, thawed

1/4 teaspoon dried oregano

1/4 teaspoon dried basil

6 ounces fettuccine, cooked and drained

Instructions

1. Whisk together ricotta cheese and milk; put aside. Take an outsized skillet, heat oil over medium heat. Add garlic and

pepper; sauté 1 minute. Add subsequent seven ingredients. Cook and blend over medium heat until vegetables are crisp tender, about 5 minutes.

2. Add cheese mixture to fettuccine; top with vegetables. Toss to coat. Serve immediately.

Nutrition

229 calories, 7g fat (3g saturated fat), 13mg cholesterol, 88mg sodium, 31g carbohydrate (6g sugars, 4g fibre), 11g protein.

Bow Ties with Sausage & Asparagus

Ingredients

3 cups of uncooked whole wheat bow tie pasta (about 8 ounces)

1 pound of asparagus, cut into 1-1/2-inch pieces

One package (19-1/2 ounces) Italian turkey sausage links, casings removed

One medium onion, chopped

Three garlic cloves, minced

1/4 cup shredded Parmesan cheese

Additional shredded Parmesan cheese, optional

Instructions

1. In a 6-qt. Stockpot, prepare dinner pasta in line with package directions, including asparagus over the last 2-three minutes of cooking. Drain, reserving half cup pasta water; return pasta and asparagus to the pot.

2. Meanwhile, during a big skillet, cook sausage, onion and garlic over medium heat until no pink, 6-8 minutes, breaking sausage into large crumbles. increase stockpot. Stir in 1/four cup cheese and reserved pasta water as desired. Serve with additional cheese if desired.

Nutrition

247 calories, 7g fat (2g saturated fat), 36mg cholesterol, 441mg sodium, 28g carbohydrate (2g sugars, 4g fibre), 17g protein

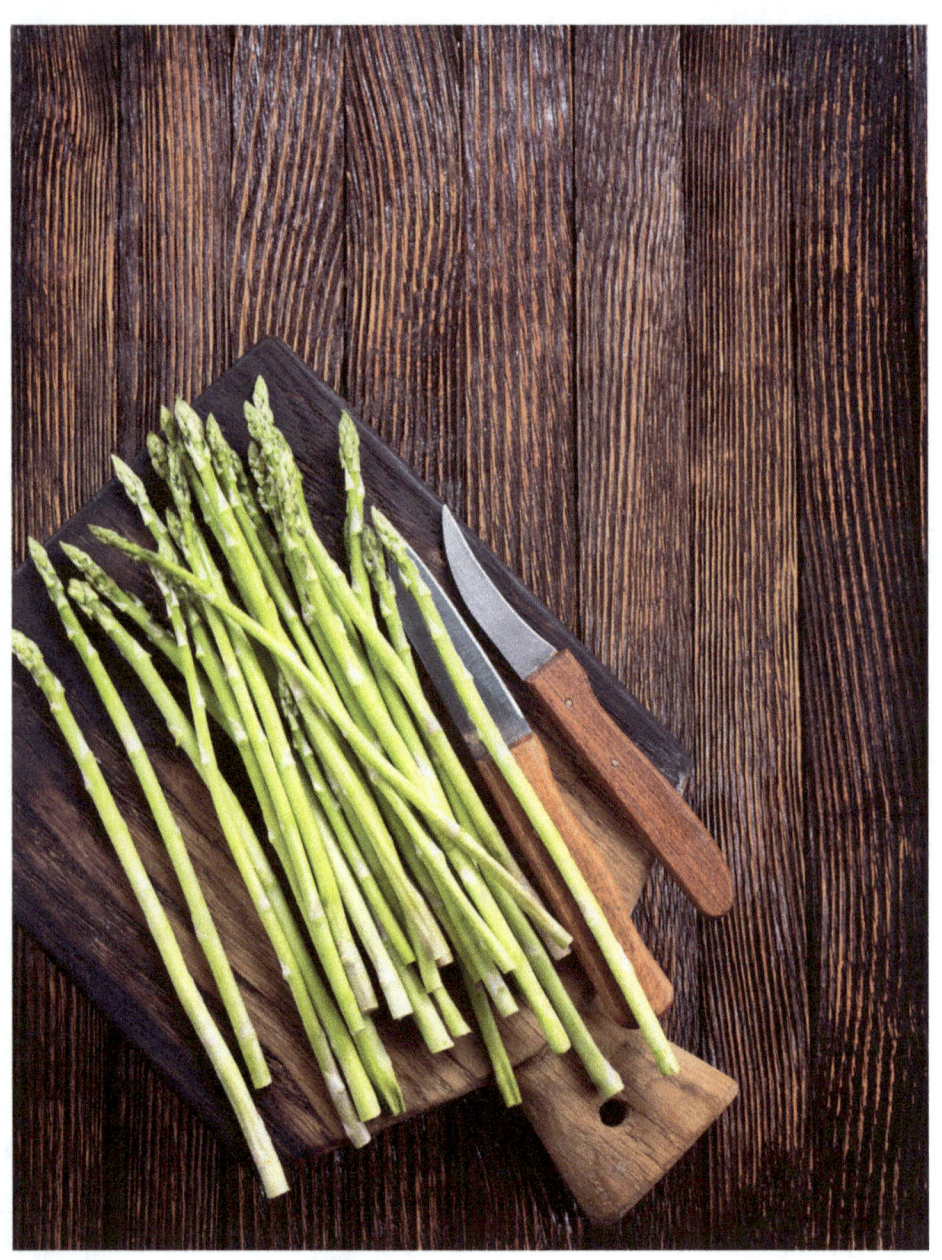

www.ingramcontent.com/pod-product-compliance
Lightning Source LLC
Chambersburg PA
CBHW070732030426
42336CB00013B/1948